Dennis Moeck
Illustrated by **Ulrike Annyma Kern**

Essential Oils
ORACLE CARDS

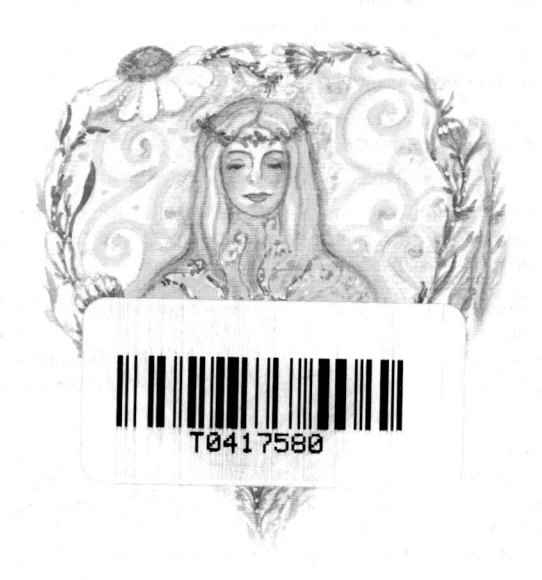

*Wisdom and Guidance
from 40 Healing Plants*

Great care has gone into writing and checking the advice in this card set. However, it does not represent a substitute for expert medical consultation and so should be used in conjunction with, and to stimulate, your own powers of self-healing. It is provided with no express or implicit guarantee on the part of the author or publisher. The author and the publisher and its agents cannot accept any liability for any injury to persons or loss or damage to property.

First edition 2023
Essential Oils Oracle Cards
Wisdom and Guidance from 40 Healing Plants
Dennis Moeck
Illustrated by Ulrike Annyma Kern

First English edition © 2023 Earthdancer GmbH
English translation © 2023 JMS books LLP
Editing by JMS books LLP (www.jmseditorial.com)

Originally published in German as: *Die Heilkraft der Pflanzenseelen, Weisheits-Orakel der ätherischen Öle und Pflanzen*
World © 2021 Schirner Verlag, Darmstadt, Germany

All rights reserved. No part of this book may be reprinted or reproduced or utilized in any form or by any electronic, mechanical, or other means, now known or hereafter invented, including photocopying and recording, or in any information storage or retrieval system, without permission in writing from the publisher.

Design and typography:
DesignIsIdentity.com
Box and book jacket background:
Nik Merkulov/shutterstock.com
Printed and bound in China by Reliance Printing Co. Ltd.

MIX
Paper from responsible sources
FSC® C102842

ISBN 978-1-64411-879-5

Published by Earthdancer, an imprint of Inner Traditions
www.earthdancerbooks.com, www.innertraditions.com

Dedication

We dedicate this card set to our female ancestors, our earthly mothers in heaven, Mother Nature, the mother of all healing plant souls, and Mother Earth, the divine mother. You gave us life, taught us, and guided us, for which we feel the deepest gratitude and love!

For you, Mother! Thank you for always being in my heart and for filling it with your love and belief in me.

Dennis Moeck

In love and gratitude for my mother, Sigrid Wilke, who was my teacher and a wonderful artist.

Ulrike Annyma Kern

How we discovered the healing souls of plants

For a long time we have been fascinated by the fragrance of precious incense and exquisite essential oils. A few years ago, when I (Dennis) encountered what for me is the purest of essential oils, vibrating at the very highest of frequencies, it was as if stories, old memories, and entities were being revealed to me through their use. They became my daily companions and my teachers. I came to understand that all things that live, thrive, and survive have an aura, a link to the morphic field (which is connected to everything that is, so any information can be retrieved from it) and as such are able to communicate with each other. Included in these are the healing souls of plants, which are more similar to humans than we might at first think. I have undergone great transformations within myself through the routine use and application of oils, healing emotional hurt and also achieving progress of which I had never dared dream. I have also made use of these intriguing aromas in my work with others, enjoying experiences that I have recorded, and, through my contact with the souls of plants, traveling to places in my inner world that have awakened a calling within me. This calling is to share the emotional and spiritual healing power of the souls of plants with the world.

This feeling of a purpose gradually grew within me over the course of some three years until, on one particular evening, I drew a card from Ulrike Annyma Kern's universal healing set (*Heilerkarten: Botschaften aus dem universellen Heilungsfeld*, published in 2019 by Schirner

Verlag) and, in a flash, I had a revelation, an insight into the way we could work together. An image came to me of how we could collaborate, and from that moment on, it was as though the souls of plants themselves were leading the way. Ulrike and I both experienced a deep spiritual memory through each other. Together, we "saw" images that she then transposed with artistic clarity and high frequency vibrations. As we worked on the cards, we were guided toward our own processes of healing and transformation, and we let this powerful aura flow into the cards through our words, images, and energy.

May the healing souls of plants be a blessing to us all as our constant companions and spiritual comforters. May our experiences with them be a radiant way to realize the light of all-encompassing love.

Dennis Moeck

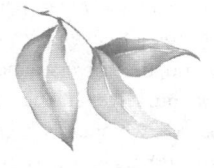

The vibration of healing plant souls

Everything that exists is animated by an all-pervading power, a power that reminds us of our divine origins, our divine unity, through which we always work when connected to it.

When we work with essential oils, we enter a subtle plane that can lead us to a higher vibration. The true soul and aura of plants is revealed to us, plants whose origins lie in the eternal space of the cosmos and which have manifested themselves on the material, earthly plane. They appear to us as archetypes—as beautiful women, as angels, masters, or sages, or as children. They give us their own talents and creativity once we become aware of their wisdom and love. Make use of this ancient gift and the healing power of the souls of plants, which all work differently for and with us and yet, on the level of the divine, are all part of a greater whole, just as we humans are.

If, with great love and mindfulness, and in harmony with all of Nature, the healing soul of a plant is distilled with all its active ingredients, its subtle forces, the spirit of each particular resin, flower, or herb will also be revealed to us. Since plants, just like humans, possess a morphic field, they are able to communicate with and reveal new paths to us. They can transform suffering and even help us to connect with the origins of the world, the universe, and the source of life.

We may immerse ourselves in the soul of a plant, and listen intently to its soft whisper as we find the wholeness of our own soul through its loving support and wisdom.

Ways in which to use the cards

Use this set of cards to:
- connect with the healing power of the souls of plants;
- work with the souls of plants in therapeutic treatments or group work;
- work with essential oils and use the cards as a kind of handbook, a reference source;
- use essential oils in conjunction with the wisdom of oracle cards;
- discover inspiration, ideas, and support through a better connection with yourself when making decisions.

Harness the power of healing plant souls intuitively for any life issue, both for yourself and for others. They will be at your side as **companions, guides, motivators,** and even as loving **mentors**. You can also use the cards in conjunction with any of your own teaching sessions or readings in order to recognize issues more clearly and to influence them in a positive manner through the symbolism of the cards and the messages they contain.

In this way, the precise healing plant soul that wants to find its way to you will always do so. The cards can be used to boost the energy of a room or as a constant reminder of the subtle vibration of plants.

On the face of each card (in landscape format), you will find a **symbolic representation** of each plant soul, which, as you gaze at it, instantly embraces you with its wisdom and love. Its message also inspires and guides, encouraging and spurring you into action. The reverse of the cards (in portrait format) features the **theme** and **affirmation** associated with each plant, which you can consult while using the relevant oil. As it takes effect, discover how the soul of the plant can work with and within you to release inner blockages, turn visions into reality, and assist with decision-making. Each card has a **top tip** on how to use the oil in your own life. I recommend that you take the trouble to read the **aspects** listed for each plant somewhere peaceful and quiet, in order to sense with your body which of the aspects you resonate with (which may vary from day to day). The higher the resonance you feel, the more effective the oil. This is a clear indication that the oil may accompany you on that particular day or over a chosen period of time. The **chakras** specified indicate in which area the soul of the plant will be particularly effective on an energetic level.

Before using the cards for the first time, I recommend that you greet them by studying them attentively and touching them one by one. This will bring you into contact with the healing plant souls. If you so wish, hold the cards over your heart and welcome them in your own words.

Before each (subsequent) use, for a powerful effect, tap on the cards three times while imagining how the energy previously generated through the cards so far is now leaving them. This will cleanse and clear cards.

How you phrase the question that you wish to ask is entirely up to you, but to ensure that any message you receive is presented clearly and in a helpful way, it is a good idea to formulate each question openly. Here are some suggestions.

- Which of my ideas and impulses are important to me today?
- Which essential oil can provide me with the most effective support today or in the coming days?
- What wisdom do I want to work with even more intensively?
- Which of my chakras may I harmonize?
- How can I support my body, mind, and spirit, and my ambitions; how can I begin a process of disengagement, or help to dispel my fear of . . . ?
- What will encourage me to take this step?

Shuffling the cards is a pleasant preliminary ritual to do while thinking about to what you need an answer, in which matter you need guidance in terms of how to react, or which course of action to take. Shuffle the cards with the representation of the plant souls face up while whispering your question or intended plan of action.

Should a card happen to fall out as you shuffle, then it is a sign and an important message! You can now either fan out the cards in front of you, with the representation of the plants souls face down, and pick a card, or close your eyes and select the top card from the pile. Depending on what kind of answer you were seeking, this card can be used as your affirmation card, which you can look at as often as you like when you feel the need to do so—every day, month, or even year, for example. Place it by your bed, on an altar, or elsewhere, with the affirmation clearly visible (and ideally next to a vial of the relevant plant oil), to remind you of the theme and the intention of the card.

To reinforce the power of the cards, use the magic of the natural oils, which you can apply after selecting an affirmation card or performing a reading, in order to fully integrate the healing plant soul with your intention. The oil can also be carried with you as an anchor scent. Use the oil as described in the **top tip** on the relevant card or apply it to the chakra specified on the card.

Classic methods of reading cards

LAYING THREE CARDS
Using your intuition, select three cards.
Card no 1: What is really at the heart of the matter? (past)
Card no 2: What should I focus on, where is the solution to be found? (present)
Card no 3: What course of action lies ahead? (future)

If you would like to work with the relevant essential oils, follow the next steps.

1. Apply the first (diluted) oil to the area over your liver in a circular motion and let go mentally. Say "I free myself from the past."

2. Apply the second (diluted) oil to your third eye (in the center of your forehead) and to the crown chakra (place a little oil in the palm of your left hand, and with the index finger of your right hand, rub the oil into the scalp on the very top of your head) to orient and balance yourself. Focus on finding the solution as you do so.

3. Apply the third (diluted) oil to the soles of your feet and massage it in, sweeping its essence into your aura as you do so. Pause for a while to sense the results, then physically walk a few steps forward as you set in motion the impulses of the future within you.

Tip
Use all three oils in a diffuser to support yourself on all levels with the power of their fragrances.

SEEKING ADVICE FROM HEALING PLANT SOULS

For this special reading, you may decide wholly intuitively how many healing plant souls you wish to consult regarding your current decision, any issues in your life, or even if there is a crisis to be resolved. It is best not to ask the advice of too many plant souls at once, however.

Working with one card
Shuffle the cards, pick one, and place it in front of you. Connect with the soul of the plant depicted and tell it what is currently on your mind, causing you concern, or where you seek spiritual support.

Imagine that you are integrating with the energy of the healing plant soul and look back at yourself. Sense yourself as a powerful plant in all your grace, beauty, and love. What advice do you give yourself? It might be to use your intuition, or you might discover an inner message, or some kind of trigger or impulse to do something.

Return to your own self, breathe deeply, absorb the advice, and then take a couple of minutes to reflect on it. Are there any other issues where the soul of the plant can deliver support? In this way, by changing roles and switching places with a plant, however many times it takes, you can make a connection and seek the plant's advice.

Work with this same essential oil for the next 21 days and be open and receptive to all the messages it may bring you.

Working with several cards
If you have selected several souls of plants, imagine yourself slipping into each of them and examine your issue from a range of different spiritual viewpoints. Once you have done this, or even while doing it, if you have the oils to hand, you may like to make a roll-on or diffuser mixture that can provide additional support for the next 21 days. For the roll-on mixture, fill an empty glass container with a carrier oil and add four or five drops of each essential

oil. Keep it with you at all times and apply the mix of oils to your wrists, temples (be careful with the hot oils such as cinnamon!), or over your heart space.

Working with essential oils, safety information

This information relates to pure essential oils. See also any safety advice provided on the labels of the bottles.

Essential oils can often be applied undiluted to the palms of the hands and the soles of the feet. However, when applied to other parts of the skin, they need to be diluted with a carrier oil (almond, coconut, or jojoba oil). Test oils such as lavender, frankincense, or copaiba on the skin on the inside of the elbow to see if any irritation occurs. If there is no sign of irritation or reaction, they can often also be applied undiluted, but always take care and follow the instructions on the label.

It is important to remember the following.

- Always have a pure, plant-based oil to hand to "erase" and/or rinse off an essential oil in the event that it causes a rash or some form of irritation.
- Never allow oil to enter the eyes. If some oil does find its way into the eye, rinsing with a carrier oil can help. Note: Water only intensifies the burning sensation.
- Pure citrus oils are considered photosensitive and so may increase the effects of sunlight. If skin treated with undiluted essential oil is then exposed to direct sunlight

or UV light within 72 hours, it can cause a reaction to, or pigmentation of, the skin.
- Essential oils with high levels of menthol (such as peppermint and eucalyptus) should not be used on children under the age of three. In the case of peppermint, this also applies to nursing mothers, as the oil can pass to the infant via the mother's milk.
- The following oils should not be used during pregnancy: basil, sage, fennel, hyssop, eucalyptus, jasmine, chamomile, marjoram, myrrh, cloves, oregano, rosemary, thyme, and cinnamon.
- Discuss the use of essential oils with your doctor if you have any allergies, irritations, or conditions associated with medication.

The author

Dennis Moeck is a qualified mind coach and successful blogger. He offers individual sessions, online courses, and also training programs. He organizes retreats and workshops on such topics as *Journeying to inner worlds*, *Changing consciousness*, *Ayurveda*, *Modern rituals*, and *Aromatherapy*. He has been working intensively with crystals and essential oils for many years.

The artist

Ulrike Annyma Kern is an artist, author, and teacher of wisdom, and has been accompanying people on their spiritual journeys for more than 15 years. She teaches the essence and the effects of universal, divine energies in her books, card sets, and artwork, together with her seminars and training courses. She lives and works in Herborn in the German state of Hesse, where she helps people to recognize their true selves and bring the light of their souls' essence into the world.

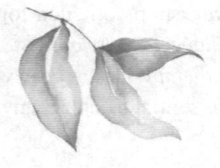

For further information and to request a book catalogue contact:
Inner Traditions, One Park Street, Rochester, Vermont 05767

Earthdancer Books is an Inner Traditions imprint.
Phone: +1-800-246-8648, customerservice@innertraditions.com
www.earthdancerbooks.com • www.innertraditions.com

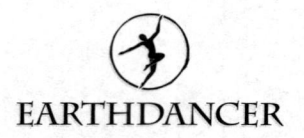

EARTHDANCER

AN INNER TRADITIONS IMPRINT